PALEO SMOOTHIES

Healthy Smoothie Recipes Book with Over 60 Nutritious
Paleo Fruit, Vegetable, Protein and Dairy Free Smoothies

by Jane Burton

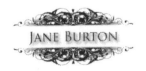

© 2015 by Jane Burton
Published by Kangaroo Flat Books

ISBN - 978-0-9925435-6-3

ISBN -10: 0992543568

Visit the Author's Page

for the full color, linked Kindle or PC book format.

www.amazon.com/author/janeburton

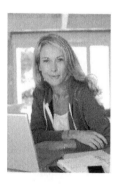

Table of Contents

WHY SMOOTHIES?

Before we begin, I would like to thank you for buying this book. I hope you enjoy it!

A quick look at the Paleo diet, also known as the Caveman diet, encourages an old-school approach to eating. It encompasses the best characteristics about dieting and nutrition. It's a high protein, low glycemic diet which is perhaps the best way to lose weight and stay healthy...long term. It's also very high in fruits and vegetable that contain high amounts of healthy vitamins and minerals. Another benefit is a good intake of omega 3 fatty acids which help calm inflammation in the body. The idea is to change your eating habits so that you eat a diet consisting of very natural or unrefined foods to boost your health and metabolism. This will in turn give you more energy and help you to trim down and lose weight. It's quite an easy diet to follow with the key Paleo food rule being - if it is NOT natural, it's out. Meats, fruits and vegetables must be unprocessed and preservative free.

Nutritionally, breakfast is regarded to be the most important meal of the day and yet countless people skip it; including children! Whether it's because facing food first thing in the morning isn't your thing or that you just don't have enough time to make breakfast, a simple solution is making smoothies. Smoothies are not only a quick and easy way to eat a nutritious meal when you are busy, but they also offer a tasty, refreshing drink. If you follow the Paleo diet, these healthy smoothie recipes will fit right into your lifestyle.

We love making smoothies at our house because they are so flexible with ingredients. They can also save you money if you buy fruits or vegetables on special at the supermarket, or if you have an abundance from your own garden. Of course when people are on their way to work or kids are off to school, smoothies are a perfect quick to prepare choice. Paleo smoothies don't differ all that much from regular fruit or vegetable smoothies, but they probably differ the most when it comes to their dairy content. The recipes in this book are all dairy free. Some recipes call for almond milk or coconut milk instead. Smoothies are great for weight loss being full of fibre, vitamins and minerals. Some people find them useful for fasting or as a meal replacement.

These easy to make, nourishing Paleo smoothies are great for adults and kids of all ages. You can play around with many of the ingredients and come up with your own favorites. You can leave things out or add some new ones if you prefer a particular taste. That's what I love about them, they are so changeable but still so tasty and nutritious. Change things up and try something new. Have fun, be creative!

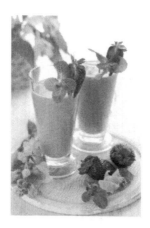

7 Good Reasons for Making Smoothies!

Healthy smoothies benefit our bodies and our lives in numerous ways.

- Rich in nutrients, vitamins and oils
- Contains healthy dietary fat required for burning energy and healthy biological functions
- Assists with keeping the body hydrated
- Assists in weight loss and even healthy meal replacement
- Preparation, consumption and digestion are simple
- Constipation can be a thing of the past!
- Healthy all-in-one quick Paleo meal when you are busy!

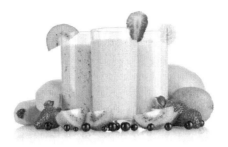

Smoothie Tips

Start the morning with a delicious fresh fruit breakfast smoothie that's not only loaded with vitamins, antioxidants, healthy fats and protein but tastes amazing! Use fruits that are in season. These will not only save you money, but taste a lot better too.

Remember, if the ingredients are wilting or not ripe, the taste will be compromised. If you have a powerful blender, you can even add a few dried fruits, dark chocolate, nuts and seeds to many of these recipes.

Purchase organic fruits, or locally grown if possible. Following Paleo means natural in every aspect where possible, so chemical laced ingredients are to be avoided. Wash or peel the fruits and vegetables first.

You will need a decent sized, powerful blender or food processor for harder vegetables or fruits. Adding chia seeds and flaxseed oils are great for your health too. If you struggle to purchase fresh produce, then you may need to add some canned fruits or vegetables, or some vanilla extract. If honey isn't mixing into your smoothie properly, then try gently warming it first to make it runny in consistency.

When using kale, broccoli or other harder type fruit or vegetable, try removing the stringy tough stems or better still lightly steam the whole thing to get all the nutrient benefit. If you have a powerful machine, this won't be such a problem.

If you have leftovers, freeze them into ice cubes for later, or make them into popsicles!

www.amazon.com/author/janeburton

30 SMOOTHIE DETOX SUPER FOODS

While many fruits and vegetables have a variety of helpful effects on our bodies, this is just a snapshot of a few and some of the benefits they hold. Try to incorporate these into your smoothies wherever possible. This list comes from my Juicer Recipes book.

- Natural protein boosters for weight gain and vitality include egg yolk, natural nut butters, ground nuts and seeds, coconut & almond milks. Don't forget, using your muscles builds muscle!
- Cabbage juice is good for the stomach and treating peptic ulcers.
- Leafy green vegetable juice can help it treating leg ulcers and sores.
- Beets are good for cleansing the liver, gall bladder and bowel.
- Natural sweeteners can be used such as soaked dates, raisins, and prunes. Date sugar, maple syrup, carob powder and raw honey are also good.
- Apple and pineapple juice are good to help cover up a "yucky" taste.
- Cayenne pepper is good for circulation.
- Alfalfa is good for bowel health.
- Anise (herb) will help reduce gas in the stomach.
- Citrus fruits, and any fruit/veg high in ascorbic acid help boost the immune system and fight cancer.
- Carrots contain beta carotene which help fight infection and cancer.
- Coriander (cilantro) is good for the heart and the digestive system.
- Dandelion is a mild diuretic.
- Echinacea is a good detoxifying agent for cleaning the lymphatic system.
- Figs and prunes are a natural laxative
- Grapes are a good blood purifier.
- Kale is high in calcium and good for our teeth and bones.
- Lemons, oranges and grapefruit help eliminate catarrh, and boost immune system.
- Flaxseed and nut oils have Omega 3.

- Mangoes are good for the intestines.
- Almond milk and almond milk is a good source of protein.
- Lettuce can slow digestion, but is good for insomnia.
- Parsley is a tonic for the kidneys and blood vessels.
- Mint is good to help cover a "yucky" taste and also good for digestion.
- Pineapple is a good source of manganese and vitamin C, great for the blood and digestion.
- Pomegranate is good for urinary problems and is a detox blood cleanser.
- Papaya is good for intestinal disorders.
- Radish is good for catarrh.
- Sage is a good "wake up" herb and also good for the sinuses.
- Spinach is great raw in drinks, but don't overdo it because it contains oxalic acid.
- Thyme helps alleviate headaches, asthma and cold symptoms associated with the upper respiratory system.
- Watermelon is good for the kidneys and is a blood cooler.
- Watercress helps eliminate fluids from the body because it is high in potassium.
- Wheatgrass is high in Indole which helps prevent cancer. It is high in many beneficial enzymes.

Kale Smoothie

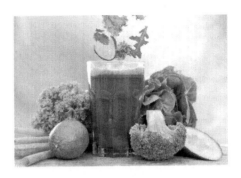

Ingredients:

1 ripe pear - (cored & cut into chunk size pieces)

1-2 cups seedless grapes of your choice

1 cups washed kale leaves, tough white stems removed if prefer

1 cup broccoli florets or kale (lightly steamed to reduce hardness)

1 cup coconut cream (coconut milk works too)

1 cup apple juice

juice of half a lime (optional)

Directions:

Place all ingredients in a blender & puree until smooth. Serve immediately.(serves 3-4) The combination of green veggies and fresh fruit for lots of health-promoting goodness!

Orange Sunrise Smoothie

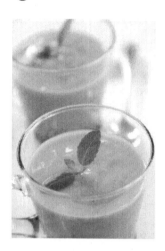

Ingredients:

1 ½ cups almond milk

1 cup mango, cut into cubes (or honeydew melon)

1 banana, peeled

1 seedless orange, peeled and divided in sections

shredded coconut for garnish (optional)

Directions:

Pour the almond milk in the blender, then add all the other ingredients except the coconut shreds. Blend until smooth and mango is well incorporated. Pour into glasses and garnish with the coconut shreds.

The Hangover Smoothie

This smoothie is a great "pick me up" when you are sick and don't really feel like eating, but need something nutritious. This will be good for energy levels, even if they only drink half of it and put the rest in the fridge for later...or freeze it.

Ingredients:

1 cup pineapple juice

1/2 cup almond milk

1 cup strawberries, fresh or frozen (berries help detox the liver)

1/4 cup peach slices with or without skin (if you don't want it too sweet, use a banana for nutrient rich potassium)

2 tspn of flax oil

1 Tbsp agave nectar, honey or maple syrup

1 - 2 Tbsp almond meal (almonds are good for nausea)

1/2 tspn diced ginger (optional, but it is good for nausea)

Directions:

Blend up all together until smooth. Drink what you can and put the rest in the fridge.

Fruit & Vegetable Wash Recipe

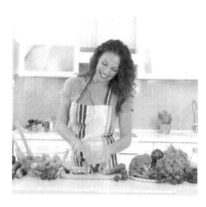

You will need to wash your fruits and vegetables if they aren't organic to remove any chemical residue or dirt that may be lingering. This is why home grown veggies, herbs and fruits are so good - you don't have to worry about quality control!

Ingredients:

1 cup vinegar
1 cup water
2 Tbsp lemon juice
1 Tbsp baking soda

Directions:

Place all ingredients into a large bowl and mix together. After all the fizzing from the baking soda is finished, pour the mix into a spray bottle. Spray your produce and leave it stand for at least a few minutes before washing off thoroughly.

BLENDED SMOOTHIE JUICES

There are so many different types on juicing machines on the market these days, the blending, juicing and smoothie options are limitless. Some blend everything up as a smoothie, while some juicers remove the pulp from just about anything. It gets down to how old your machine is and the different functions is has available. Of course the top end machines come at a price.

It's possible to blend together a smoothie style mix and juicer mix if that is what it takes to make a healthy, tasty drink! You can be adventurous; experiment, as many favorite Paleo smoothies are born this way!

The other great thing about mixing blended drinks together is you get the best of both worlds by adding healthy ingredients you wouldn't normally be able to put into a smoothie. They help make a natural super food in a glass! If you are interested in Juicer recipes check out my book. So be creative and try creating your own health drinks by using what you have handy. Variety is the spice of life!

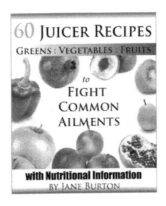

Paleo Pumpkin Perfection

Ingredients:

1/2 cup of pumpkin puree

1 tspn mixed spice (or cinnamon)

1/2 tspn vanilla extract

3/4 cup unsweetened coconut milk

1 chilled or frozen banana

6-7 ice cubes

honey to taste (I use about 2 tspn)

Directions:

Blender until smooth. Garnish with mint and some nutmeg if desired.

Iced Coffee Frappe

Ingredients:

2 Tbsp raw honey (mix this into the coffee while still warm)

1 cup good quality brewed coffee, chilled

1/4 cup coconut cream (from the top)

1/2 tspn vanilla extract

1 heaped Tbsp 100% cocao powder

Directions:

Make the coffee, add the honey, then chill. Blend all ingredients together.

Classic Breakfast Smoothie

Smoothies are perfect for breakfasts because they are easy to make and full of vitamins. They only take minutes to prepare, need minimal cleanup and equate to a fast meal in a glass...Fabulous when you are trying to watch your health and watch the time on a busy morning!

Ingredients:

1 cup of strawberries

½ cup of blueberries

½ cup water

1 banana, mashed

1 egg

4-5 ice cubes

Directions:

Blend all ingredients until smooth. Very flexible, use fruits you have on hand.

Strawberry Bliss Smoothie

Ingredients:

1 cup fresh water

6 big strawberries, stems removed

1 seedless orange, peeled and divided into sections

1 mango, cut into cubes

1 banana, peeled

6 ice cubes

Directions:

Place all ingredients in blender and blend for a couple of minutes until smooth. Pour the smoothie in glasses and serve.

Black Forrest Smoothie

Simple, pure bliss.

Ingredients:

1 cup coconut milk (almond milk works too)

1 - 1 1/2 cups pitted, canned dark Morello cherries or other fresh cherries

2 Tbsp unsweetened 100% cocoa powder

1/2 small banana

Directions:

Blend it all up. Sprinkle with grated natural dark chocolate and shredded coconut if desired.

Emerald Smoothie

A monster for nutrition!

Ingredients:

1 cup coconut milk

1 cup kale, stems removed

1 cup baby spinach leaves, washed

½ cup mango, cut into cubes

1 banana, peeled

1/2 tspn chia seeds (optional)

½ cup water

½ cup ice cubes

1 tspn honey if you wish to have a sweeter smoothie

Directions:

Pour the coconut milk in the blender, then add all the other ingredients. Blend until smooth. Garnish with a baby spinach leaf or halved strawberry for color.

Energizing Breakfast Smoothie

Ingredients:

1 cup coconut water

1 cup blackberries

1 cup blueberries

½ cup coconut milk (almond milk works too)

½ banana, peeled (optional)

2 Tbsp flax powder (2 tspn flaxseed oil works too)

3 tspn chia seeds

Directions:

Place all ingredients except the chia seeds in blender and blend for a couple of minutes until smooth. Stir in chia seeds. Serve and drink to your health!

Green Kale Smoothie

Have for breakfast, lunch or in the lunch box for kids or at work! This recipe comes from my allergy free, natural foods, lunch box recipes book on Amazon.

Ingredients:

1 cup fresh kale or baby spinach, washed

1 mangoes or 2 apples (for sweetness)

1 banana, peeled and chopped

juice from 1/2 a lemon or lime

1 kiwifruit, peeled and chopped

*Can add 1 tspn chia seeds and 1 tspn flaxseed oil.

Directions:

1. *Process all ingredients in a blender until well mixed. Pour into sealed cups/containers and refrigerate.*

If you partially freeze, this can be used as a chiller pack to keep lunches cool. Simple, healthy and delicious!

Cashew and Date Shake

Ingredients:

1/2 cup cold coconut milk or coconut cream

1/4 cup raw unsalted cashews, soaked for about 6 - 8 hours until softened

1 tspn chia seeds (optional)

1/2 banana

2 - 3 pitted Medjool dates (adjust to your taste)

about 4 ice cubes

Directions:

In a small container, soak the cashews in the milk or cream and cover. When ready to make the smoothie, blend it all together really well to get a smooth consistency.

Carrot Cake Smoothie

Ingredients:

1 chilled or frozen banana

1 cup chopped carrots

1 cup coconut cream

1/4 cup crushed walnuts

1/3 cup unsweetened almond milk

1 Tbsp chia seeds

1/2 tspn vanilla extract

1/2 tspn cinnamon

1/2 tspn mixed spice

*1 egg optional

Directions:

Blend the first 4 ingredients all up together first, mixing well. Then add the remaining ingredients. Add more milk if you prefer.

Hearty Breakfast Smoothie

Ingredients:

2 cups frozen berries of your choice

1 cup coconut milk or cream

2/3 cup shredded coconut

1-2 eggs

Directions:

Place the berries in your blender and pulse them with a dash of hot water to break them easily. Add the coconut shreds, eggs and coconut milk. Blend until smooth. Divide the smoothie into two glasses Bottoms up!

Kiwi-Banana Breakfast Smoothie

Ingredients:

1 cup crushed ice

3 kiwi, peeled and cut into big chunks

3 bananas, cut into big chunks

1 Tbsp honey

Directions:

In a blender combine all ingredients but ice until smooth. Add ice and pulse until the smoothie is done. Pour in chilled glasses

Refreshing Green Tea Smoothie

Ingredients:

¾ cup strong brewed green tea

¼ cup almond milk

1 frozen banana

½ honeydew melon cut into big chunks

1 tspn honey

Directions:

Blend all ingredients until smooth. Pour the smoothie into glasses.

Berry Charged Energy Booster

This recipe comes from my Juicer Recipes to Fight Common Ailments
Book on Amazon. Paleo perfection!

Ingredients:

1 orange, peeled and chopped

2 bananas, peeled and blended

2 Medjool dates

A large handful of Swiss chard or spinach

1 cup blackberries or raspberries (a mix of both is even better)

1/2 cup seedless grapes in season

1/2 cup strawberries

1 cup water

Directions:

*Blend the banana. Prepare the orange and push the chard through
with this. Then add the other ingredients. Mix with the banana to make
a super smoothie. This juice is a delicious heavenly energy booster!*

Paleo Peach Smoothie

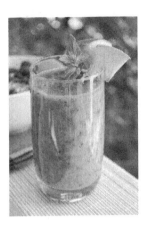

Ingredients:

3 peaches

1 banana, mashed

½ cup water

5 ice cubes

1 tspn ginger, grated

Directions:

Blend all ingredients except ice until smooth. Add ice and pulse until done. Pour the smoothie in glasses. Garnish with a sprig of mint and slice of peach.

Almond Chunky Monkey

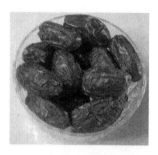

A treat on occasion. Play around to get your taste with cocoa amounts and sweetening with the dates.

Ingredients:

2 cups coconut or almond milk

1/2 Tbsp unsweetened 100% cocoa powder (or to your taste)

2 - 3 Medjool dates, or to taste

2 bananas

3 Tbsp chunky almond butter (smooth if you prefer)

Directions:

Blend on high speed in a blender until at desired consistency – smooth or chunky! May be stored in fridge for up to 2 days but will need vigorous stirring....that's if there's any left!

Egg Nog Warm Up

Strict Paleo dieters, leave out the rum!

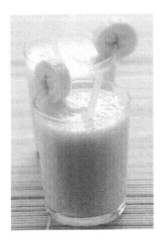

Ingredients:

1 cup coconut cream

1 large egg

1/2 tspn cinnamon

1/2 tspn nutmeg

1/4 tspn vanilla extract

dash of rum (optional)

Directions:

Blend all ingredients. Pour the smoothie into glasses topped with a sprinkle of cinnamon or sliced fruit. Serve and enjoy!

Jane Burton

Ruby Tuesday Smoothie

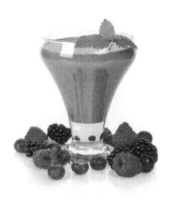

Ingredients:

1/2 cup blueberries or cranberries

1/2 cup raspberries

1 cup coconut milk (preferably chilled)

1/2 cup coconut cream (preferably chilled)

Directions:

Blend all together, very flexible with ingredients. Use what is in season.

Green Grape Surprise

Ingredients

1 cup of fresh watermelon, cut into chunks

1 orange or orange juice

1 green apple (cored & cut into small chunks)

1 peeled ripe kiwi fruit

A handful of seedless green grapes

Directions:

Blend watermelon and orange together first, then add the apple, kiwi fruit and grapes. Serve cold with a few raspberries on top. Makes 2 serves. These are great as frozen ice blocks if you have any left.

Apple Cinnamon Frappe

Serve this drink chilled.

Ingredients:

2 apples, cored and cubed (apple puree works too)

1 small banana

1 cup almond milk (unsweetened if possible)

1 Tbsp almond butter

1 tspn ground cinnamon

1 tbsp natural honey

3 ice cubes

Directions:

Blend all together until smooth. Great for breakfast! Garnish with Banana slices.

Coconut Pineapple Blast

Ingredients:

1 cup coconut milk

1 x 19oz tin unsweetened crushed pineapple (or may use fresh)

1 med banana

¼ tspn vanilla extract

Directions:

Place all ingredients in the blender, mixing until smooth.

Orange Sherbet Cocktail

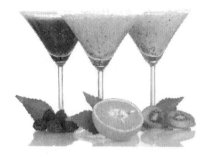

A refreshing, sparkling twist to a cool cocktail smoothie. Make them whatever color/flavor you like!

Ingredients:

1 cup chilled coconut cream

1 cup strawberries, kiwi fruit or raspberries

1½ cups fresh / tinned pineapple (drained & cut into chunks)

1½ cups chilled sparkling mineral water

1 orange, peeled, de-seeded and cubed

Directions:

Place everything into the blender; blending on high till smooth. Stir in the mineral water briskly or blend in for a few seconds only.

Banana Shake

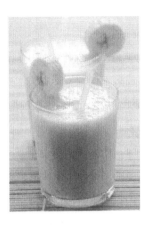

Ingredients:

2 bananas - (chopped & frozen)

3 Tbsp smooth almond butter

1 cup coconut milk

1 tspn honey

1 tspn ground hazelnuts or almonds (optional)

Directions:

Combine everything in a blender. Blend until smooth. Pop banana slices on top!

Strawberry Cream Thick Shake

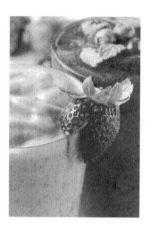

Ingredients:

8 strawberries (hulled)

1 cup coconut cream

1 - 2 Tbsp honey

2 tspn vanilla extract

6 cubes ice (crushed)

Directions:

Combine strawberries, cream, honey, vanilla and the ice last. Blend until smooth, thick and creamy. Serve with a sliced strawberry.

Energy Blaster

My son's creation before going to work.

Ingredients:

1 cup unsweetened almond milk

½ cup apple pieces

1 banana (cut into pieces)

1 small handful of fresh, washed baby spinach leaves

1 peeled carrot (cut into small pieces)

1/2 cup of fresh juice or water (optional)

1 tspn chia seeds (that's almost 2 grams of fibre!)

Directions:

Combine all ingredients in blender and blend on high till smooth. (approx. 2-3 minutes depending on blender) Garnish with a sprig of mint.

V8 Smoothie

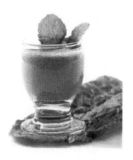

A vegetable fruit smoothie detox wonder full of energy and flavor. If you need sweetener, add some dates.

Ingredients:

1¼ cups fresh cubed mango (frozen is okay)

1 cup of chilled orange juice

1¼ cups kale leaf chunks (stems and white rib removed)

2 medium sticks of celery, chopped

¼ cup chopped flat-leaf parsley (it's more tender than the curly leaf)

¼ cup chopped fresh mint

¼ tspn ground or finely grated ginger

Directions:

Place liquids into blender, then all other ingredients and blend well.

Bloody Mary Smoothie

Okay, this one takes a little trial and error, Some like it, some hate it. Make it your own, experiment.

Ingredients:

5 ripe tomatoes, diced (the better the quality, the better the taste)

1/4 cup seeded cucumber

1 stick of celery, diced

2 - 3 Medjool dates

1 tspn natural Worcestershire sauce

1 apple

juice of one lemon

1 tspn natural horseradish (optional)

1 tspn coconut aminos

1 Tbsp vodka (strict Paleos...leave it out)

Directions:

PALEO SMOOTHIES FOR WEIGHT LOSS

When it comes to weight loss, the Paleo diet offers plenty of tasty low fat, low sugar energizing recipes. You can read more about the Paleo approach to long term healthy eating habits in my book on Amazon explaining how Paleo for Weight Loss works.

The focus in weight loss smoothies is not on the fruit, but more on vegetables, because too much fructose can actually sabotage your weight loss plans. However, there are plenty of Paleo smoothie recipes that will help you boost your metabolism while offering enough sweetness and nutrition to keep your hunger at bay. The key is getting a balance of sweet and savoury.

Sugar Count Fruit List

If you want to lose weight, let's take a look at the overall sugar content in fresh fruit. This information was gathered from the US nutrient database. Learn more about nutrients in foods at the US Nutrients Database.

Fresh Fruit: The lower the number the better, **because it has less sugar content.** You can see why berries are a popular choice when it comes to weight loss smoothies and juices; they are amongst the lowest fruit sugar count.

Apples 13.3

Apricots 9.3 1.6

Avocado 0.9

Banana 15.6

Blackberries 8.1

Blueberries 7.3

Cantaloupe 8.7

Casaba melon 4.7

Cherries, sweet 14.6

Cherries, sour 8.1

Elderberries 7

Figs 6.9

Grapefruit 6

Grapes 18.1

Guava 6

Guava, strawberry 6

Honeydew melon 8.2

Jackfruit 8.4

Kiwi fruit 10.5

Lemon 2.5

Lime 0.4

Mamey Apple 6.5

Mango 14.8

Nectarine 8.5

Orange 9.2

Papaya 5.9

Peach 8.7

Pear 10

Pineapple 11.9

Plum 7.5

Pomegranate 10.1

Passion Fruit 11.2

Raspberries 9.5

Starfruit 7.1

Strawberries 5.8

Tangerine 7.7

Tomato 2.8

Watermelon 9

Spicy Vegetable Smoothie

Ingredients:

½ cup tomato, chopped

½ cup ice

¼ cup cucumber, chopped

¼ cup raw spinach

½ avocado

2 tspn fresh lemon juice

1 tspn Paleo friendly hot sauce and/or black pepper

Directions:

Blend all ingredients and the ice until smooth. Avocado is the main source of energy in this recipe, while other ingredients provide vitamins and, of course, great taste.

Skinny Orange Freeze

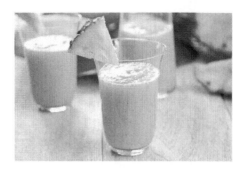

Ingredients:

1 6-oz. pack undiluted frozen orange or pineapple juice concentrate (or freshly squeezed oranges)

1 cup chilled water

1 cup unsweetened almond milk

1 tspn vanilla extract

10 ice cubes

Directions:

Add all ingredients to blender; processing until smooth. Garnish with a piece of orange or pineapple. Great in summer.

Ginger Apple Smoothie

You need to like ginger to enjoy this one!

Ingredients:

1 cup spinach

1 cup coconut water

1 cucumber, cubed

1 green apple, cored

a handful of flat leafed parsley

3 Tbsp ginger, grated

Directions:

Blend all ingredients together in your blender. If it isn't sweet enough, add 1 Tbsp honey.

Slimming Spinach Smoothie

Ingredients:

1 cup spinach leaves

3 celery stalks

2 apples, cored

1 cucumber, cut into big chunks

juice of ½ lemon

1 bunch parsley

1 tspn ginger, grated

Directions:

Combine all ingredients in the blender and blend until smooth. This one is a wonderful meal replacement.

Blueberry Kale Smoothie

Ingredients:

1 stalk kale, stem removed and chopped

½ cup frozen blueberries

¼ cup coconut water

Directions:

Blanche (boil in hot water for 1-2 minutes)the kale so it is easier to blend. Blend all ingredients ice until smooth.

Berry Slimmer

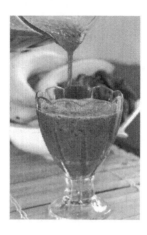

A stunning, tasty ruby wonder that's incredibly just 74 cals per serve!

Ingredients:

1½ cups boysenberry / blackberry homemade juice

1 cup boysenberries / blackberries

1 cup blueberries (fresh or frozen)

Directions:

Place all ingredients into blender & process until smooth. Absolute unadulterated heaven! Very flexible with proportions. Serve in a parfait glass for that touch of luxury!

Glowing Green Smoothie

Ingredients:

2 cups romaine lettuce, chopped

2 cups spinach, chopped

½ cup broccoli, lightly steamed and chopped

½ cup water

½ apple

½ banana

2 Tbsp fresh lemon juice

Directions:

Mix together all ingredients in a blender until smooth. Pour the smoothie in glasses. Bottoms up!

Creamy Pineapple Punch

Ingredients:

1½ cup fresh water

1 cup fresh pineapple

½ cup fennel

1 lime, peeled and seeded

½ small avocado

1 Tbsp hemp seeds

Directions:

Pulse all ingredients in the blender while slowly adding water to reach your desired consistency. Pour the smoothie in glasses.

Flat Tummy Smoothie

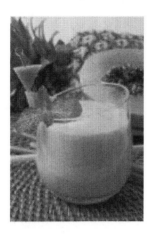

Ingredients:

1 cup water

1 cup papaya, roughly chopped

1 cup peaches, cored and roughly chopped

½ cup pear, cored and roughly chopped

2 mint leaves

1 tspn fresh ginger, grated

Directions:

Pulse all ingredients in a blender until smooth. Serve and enjoy! Add ice if you want.

Easy Tomato Veggie Smoothie

Ingredients:

2 tomatoes

3 celery ribs

1 carrot

2 Tbsp fresh lemon juice

Directions:

Combine all ingredients in a blender. Pulse until smooth. If you wish you can add a dash of hot sauce or black pepper to make this smoothie spicier. Bottoms up!

Purple Power Smoothie

Ingredients:

2 cups kale, white stems removed if preferred

2 cups blueberries

1 cup apple, cored and chopped into big chunks

1 cup water

Directions:

Blend everything in your blender until smooth.

HIGH PROTEIN SMOOTHIES

Protein is the best source of energy because it satisfies our hunger and helps us build muscle. Following Paleo guidelines, eating plenty of natural protein is encouraged as we feel full for longer and it has many benefits for our health.

The biggest problem when it comes to protein smoothies as fitness supplements or simply for energy and health, is that many of the manufactured protein shakes contain artificial protein powder that our ancestors weren't eating. However, there are plenty of healthier protein smoothie alternatives that are filling, natural and healthy. Here is a collection of such recipes.

Simple Protein Shake

Ingredients:

1 cup almond milk

3 raw eggs

2 Tbsp water

2 Tbsp honey

juice of ½ lemon

Directions:

Process all ingredients in your blender until smooth.

Banana Egg Nog Smoothie

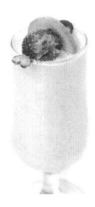

Ingredients:

1 cup coconut milk

2 egg yolks

1 frozen banana, cut in big chunks

1 tspn maple syrup

1 tspn vanilla extract

¼ tspn nutmeg

pinch of salt

Directions:

Blend egg yolks, salt and vanilla extract in a blender. Next add coconut milk and nutmeg. Add the chunks of frozen banana the last. Blend until smooth. Pour in glasses, garnish with your favorite fruits or place them on a swizzle stick. Serve and enjoy!

Avocado Twist

Avocados are low in sugar and loaded with healthy oils and nutrition. This is great if you don't feel like a particularly sweet smoothie drink.

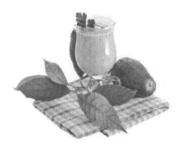

Ingredients:

1 ripe avocado
1 cup low fat milk or almond milk
2 tspn honey or maple syrup
1 basil leaf
squeeze of lime juice

Directions:

Place milk in blender, then all other ingredients and mix well. Serve chilled. Add a sprig of parsley or basil on top.

Blueberry Pumpkin Pie Smoothie

Ingredients:

1 cup almond milk

½ cup blueberries

½ cup pureed pumpkin

¼ cup walnuts

1 Tbsp cashew butter

¼ tspn cinnamon

¼ tspn nutmeg

dash of ground cloves

Directions:

Add all ingredients to a blender and process until completely combined. Pour the smoothie in glasses. Sprinkle some cinnamon over each glass for decoration.

Almond Apricot Frutti Tutti

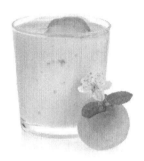

Ingredients:

2 cups almond milk

¼ cup dates

¼ cup almonds

1 banana, peeled and chopped (can use 1/2 banana 1/2 berries if desired)

1 mango, peeled and chopped in big pieces

4 fresh, seeded apricots

½ tspn vanilla extract

Directions:

Blend all ingredients in your blender until smooth. If you'd like to have greener smoothie, add one cup of spinach to the mix. Garnish with an apricot.

Chocolate Coconut Twist

Ingredients:

1 cup spinach

1 cup coconut milk

1 cup frozen berries by your choice

½ cup water

2 Tbsp coconut oil

2 Tbsp 100% cocoa powder

1 tspn cinnamon

½ tspn vanilla extract

pinch of salt

Directions:

Process all ingredients in your blender until well incorporated. Serve and enjoy the dark chocolate goodness!

Coconut Goodness

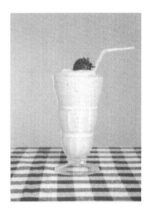

Ingredients:

2 cups chilled coconut milk

¼ cup raisins

¼ cup pumpkin seeds

1 banana, peeled and chopped

1 peach, or pear, chopped

½ tspn vanilla extract

¼ tspn cinnamon

Directions:

Blend all ingredients in your blender until smooth. Pour the smoothie into glasses and top with a strawberry.

PALEO SMOOTHIE DIET

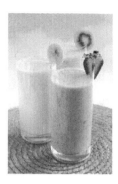

The Paleo lifestyle offers a wide variety of meal choices, and the Paleo smoothie diet is one of the many options for energizing, losing weight and feeling healthy in general. It is a good choice for vegetarians and busy people who can't spend hours in the kitchen.

People that love variety in their diet can also enjoy occasional smoothies as a meal. Here is a collection of recipes that serves that very purpose. Each smoothie is a balanced meal, so they are great as for breakfasts or light dinners.

Protein Energy Booster

Cocao nibs are highly nutritious and add crunch!

Ingredients:

1 cup almond milk

1 cup pineapple juice

½ cup raw, unsalted macadamia nuts

2 eggs

1 Tbsp cacao powder

1 tspn cocao nibs (optional)

Directions:

Whiz everything in your blender until well mixed. Pour in glasses and drink. Bottoms up!

Easy Berry Protein Smoothie

Ingredients:

1 cup grapefruit juice

1 cup mixed berries (strawberries, blueberries or any other you like)

3 egg whites

Directions:

Mix all ingredients together in a blender until smooth. Serve immediately

Mud Cake Smoothie

Ingredients:

1 cup water

12 dates, pitted

10 figs, peeled

1 Tbsp raw 100% carob powder

1 tspn cocao nibs (optional)

Directions:

Mix all ingredients until smooth. Chill and serve.

Almond Carob Smoothie

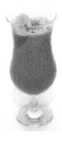

Cocao nibs are highly nutritious and add crunch!

Ingredients:

¼ cup almond milk

¼ cup almonds

1 banana, cut in big chunks

3 egg whites

1 Tbsp dried carob powder or 100% pure cocao powder

1 tspn cocao nibs (optional)

*Add some honey if you need it sweeter, or use sweetened almond milk.

Directions:

Combine all ingredients in your blender and pulse until smooth. Serve immediately with a slice of banana and enjoy!

Macadamia Smoothie

Ingredients:

1/2 cup coconut milk

1/2 cup raw macadamia nuts, soaked for about 6 hours in the coconut milk

1/2 banana, cut into chunks

1/2 tspn vanilla extract

1 dried Medjool dates, pitted

1 tspn honey (warmed slightly if it doesn't mix in)

about 6 ice cubes (optional)

Directions:

Process all ingredients in your blender until well incorporated. Last add the ice cubes. Bottoms up!

Apple Protein Drink

Ingredients:

2 cups baked apples

2 egg whites

1 tspn cinnamon

Directions:

Combine all ingredients in your blender until smooth. Chill before serving.

Nutty Green Rocket

This one packs a punch!

Ingredients:

1 cup arugula

½ cup pine nuts, soaked

1 carrot, peeled and cut in big chunks

1 sweet pepper, cut in big chunks

½ avocado, peeled and pitted

½ tomato, cut in big chunks

juice of ½ grapefruit

1 garlic clove

Directions:

Pulse all ingredients in your blender until smooth. Chill before serving. Enjoy this vegetable mix!

Strawberry Cream Delight

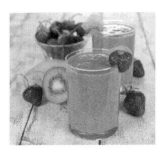

Ingredients:

1 cup strawberries (can use 1/2 cup of kiwi instead)

1/2 cup chilled coconut cream (off the top)

1/2 cup raw almonds, soaked in the coconut cream

2 chilled bananas, peeled and chopped

Directions:

Mix all ingredients until creamy. If possible, avoid adding water.

Fruity Frappe

Ingredients:

1 banana, peeled

1 orange, peeled

½ papaya, peeled

4 - 6 ice cubes

Directions:

Juice orange and papaya. Mix both juices with banana and ice in a blender until smooth. Pour in glasses and garnish with an orange twist. Serve chilled and enjoy!

Tropical Avocado Smoothie

Ingredients:

2-3 cups canned pineapple chunks (with juice)

2 cups ice

1 ripe avocado, peeled, pitted and diced

Directions:

In a blender mix together all avocado, ice and pineapple with its juice. Once all ingredients are combined, serve the smoothie.

Sweety Pie Smoothie

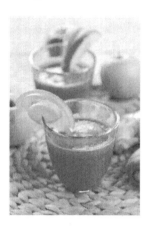

Ingredients:

1 cup strawberries

1 cup orange juice

1 carrot, scrubbed and chopped

1 apple, peeled and cored

1 pear, peeled and cored

4 ice cubes

Directions:

Whiz all ingredients in your blender until smooth. This is thick so you can freeze it into popsicles if you like or add some almond milk or water.

Other Goods Reads

Now we have the smoothies covered...you can check out my other Paleo Recipe Books on my author's page.

I hope you enjoyed this book. Reviews are an author's best friend, so if you can spare the time to leave feedback that would be much appreciated. Thank you.

- Learn more about nutrients in foods at the US Nutrients Database.
- "Low Sugar Recipes" by Peggy Annear on Amazon.

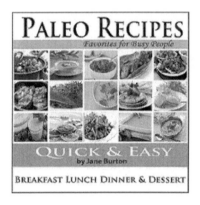

Paleo Recipes for Busy People

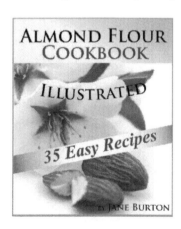

Paleo Almond Flour Recipes

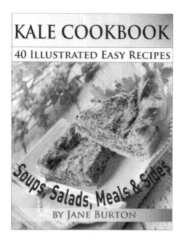

Kale Cookbook

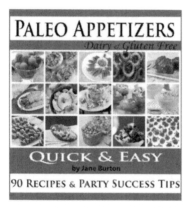

Paleo Appetizer Recipes

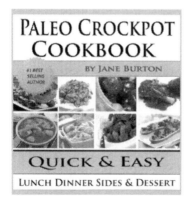

Paleo Crockpot Cookbook

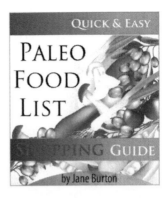

Paleo Food List & Shopping Guide

The End

Notes

Copyright

Paleo Smoothies: Copyright © 2015 by Jane Burton

Printed in Great Britain
by Amazon